MW01474236

Why We Eat Vegetables

by Beth Bence Reinke, MS, RD

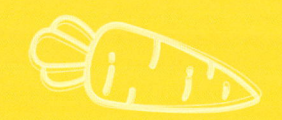

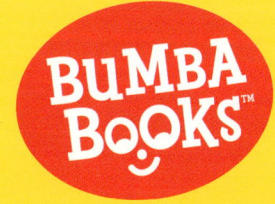

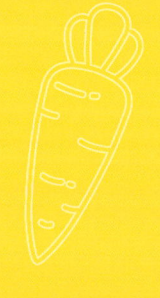

BUMBA BOOKS™

LERNER PUBLICATIONS ◆ MINNEAPOLIS

Note to Educators:

Throughout this book, you'll find critical thinking questions. These can be used to engage young readers in thinking critically about the topic and in using the text and photos to do so.

Copyright © 2019 by Lerner Publishing Group, Inc.

All rights reserved. International copyright secured. No part of this book may be reproduced, stored in a retrieval system, or transmitted in any form or by any means—electronic, mechanical, photocopying, recording, or otherwise—without the prior written permission of Lerner Publishing Group, Inc., except for the inclusion of brief quotations in an acknowledged review.

Lerner Publications Company
A division of Lerner Publishing Group, Inc.
241 First Avenue North
Minneapolis, MN 55401 USA

For reading levels and more information, look up this title at www.lernerbooks.com.

Library of Congress Cataloging-in-Publication Data

Names: Reinke, Beth Bence, author.
Title: Why we eat vegetables / Beth Bence Reinke, MS, RD.
Description: Minneapolis : Lerner Publications, [2018] | Series: Bumba books. Nutrition matters | Audience: Ages 4–7. | Audience: K to grade 3. | Includes bibliographical references and index.
Identifiers: LCCN 2017058943 (print) | LCCN 2017050329 (ebook) | ISBN 9781541507746 (eb pdf) | ISBN 9781541503366 (lb : alk. paper) | ISBN 9781541526860 (pb : alk. paper)
Subjects: LCSH: Vegetables in human nutrition—Juvenile literature. | Vegetables—Juvenile literature. | Nutrition—Juvenile literature.
Classification: LCC QP144.V44 (print) | LCC QP144.V44 R45 2018 (ebook) | DDC 613.2/8—dc23

LC record available at https://lccn.loc.gov/2017058943

Manufactured in the United States of America
1 – CG – 7/15/18

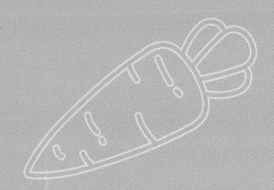

Table of Contents

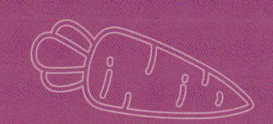

All about Vegetables 4

USDA MyPlate Diagram 22

Picture Glossary 23

Read More 24

Index 24

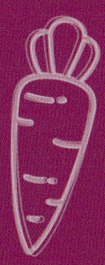

All about Vegetables

Crunch! Vegetables taste great.

They help make you strong too.

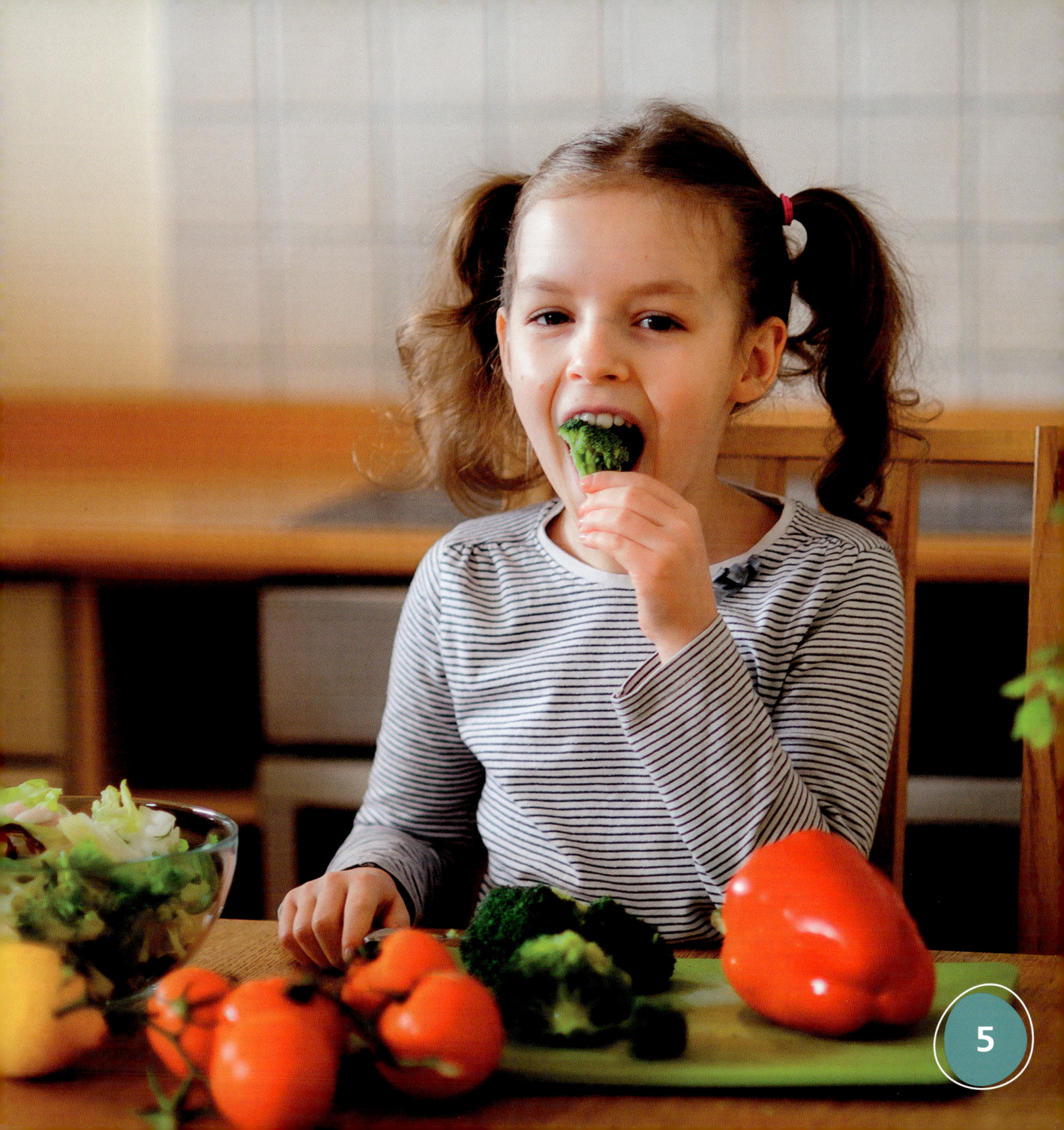

6

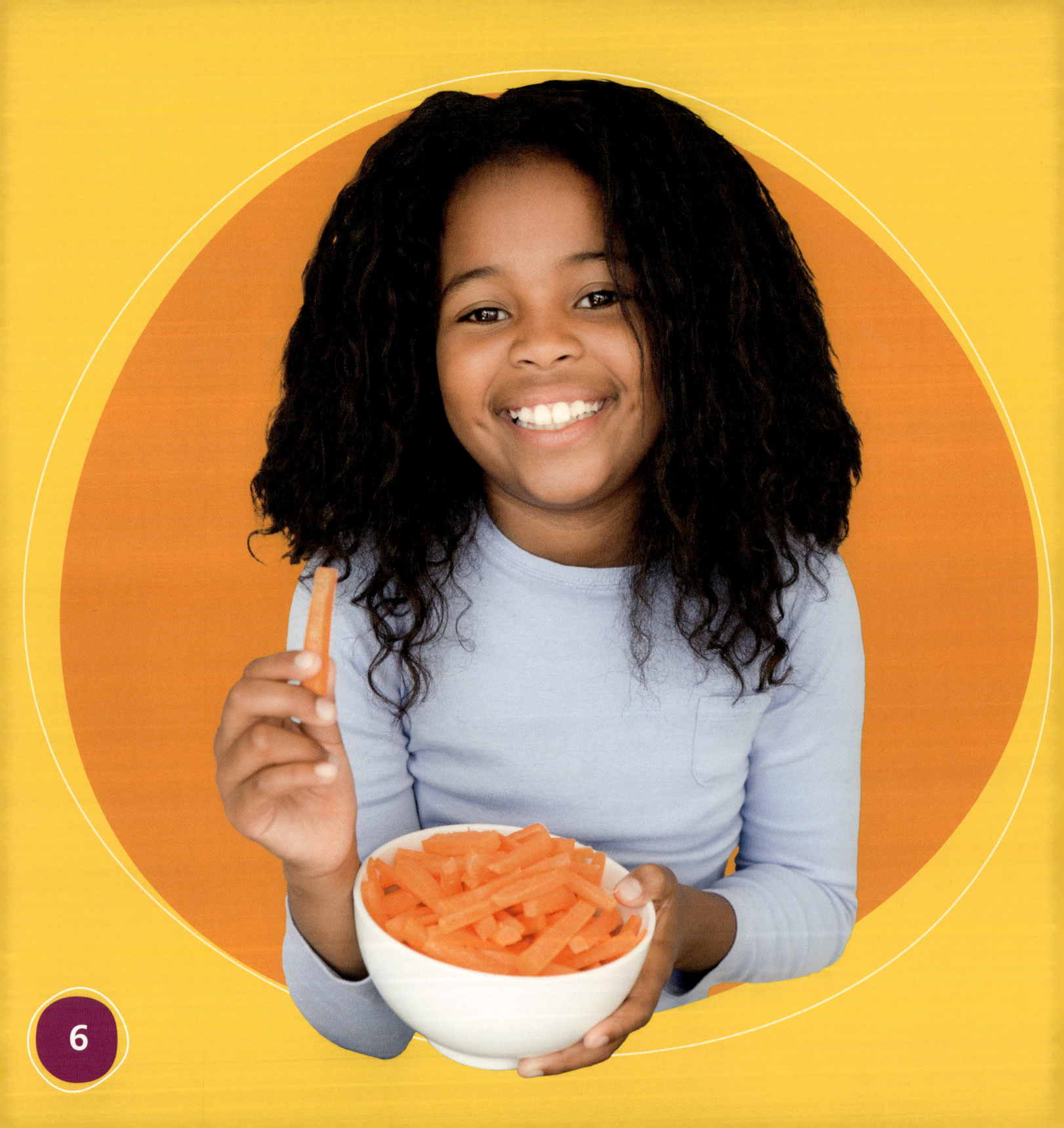

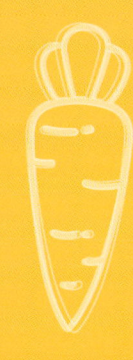

Orange vegetables give you vitamin A.

Vitamin A keeps your eyes healthy.

Can you name some orange vegetables?

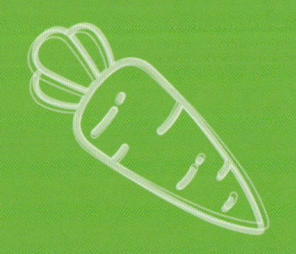

Leafy green vegetables have vitamin K. You need vitamin K for healthy bones.

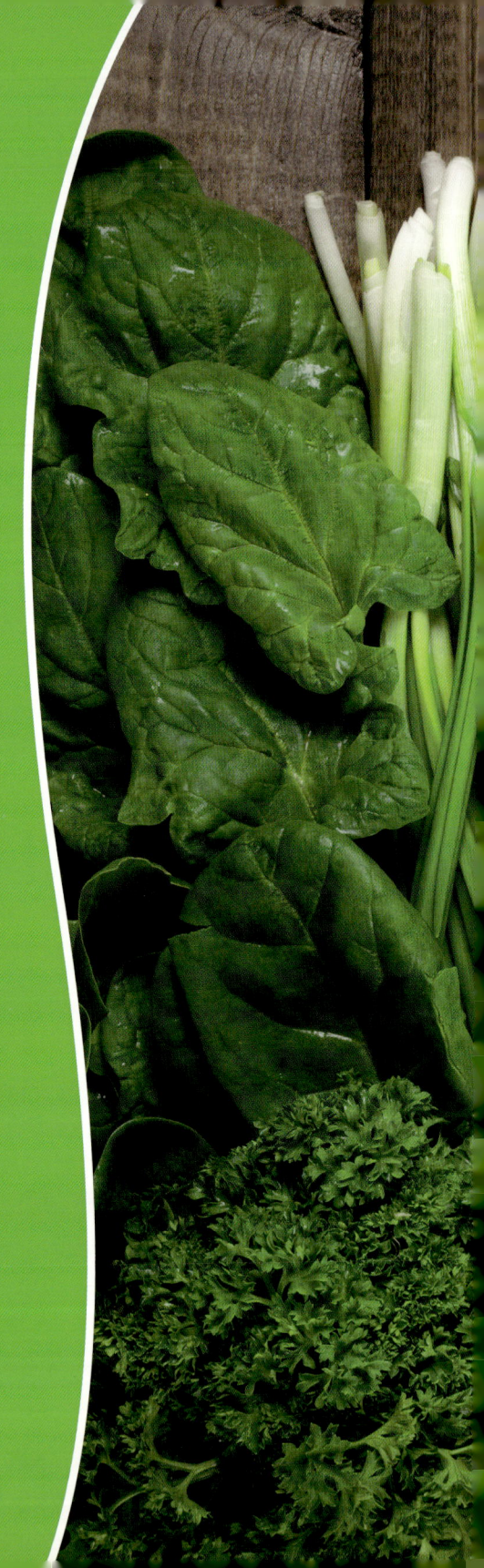

9

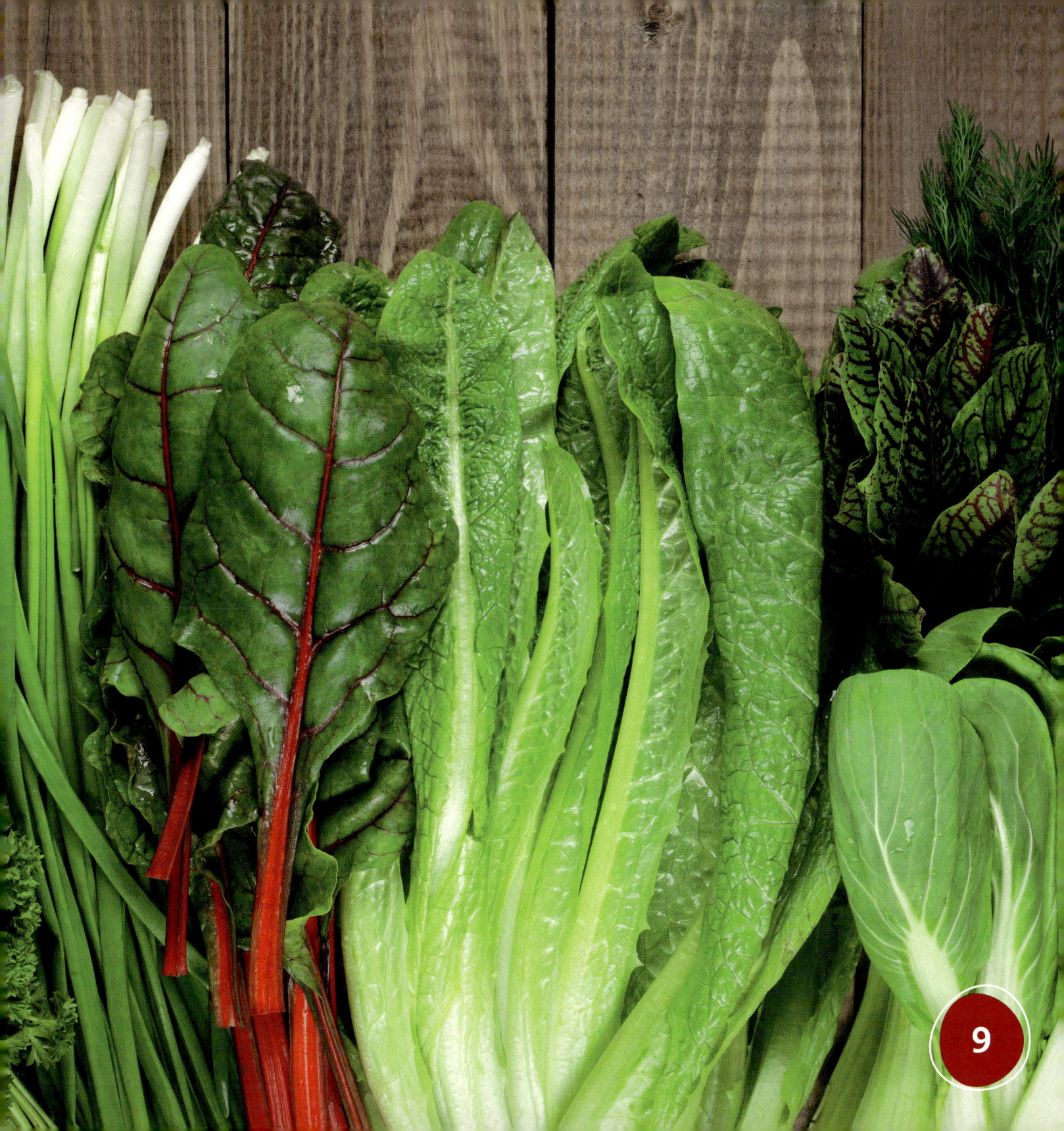

10

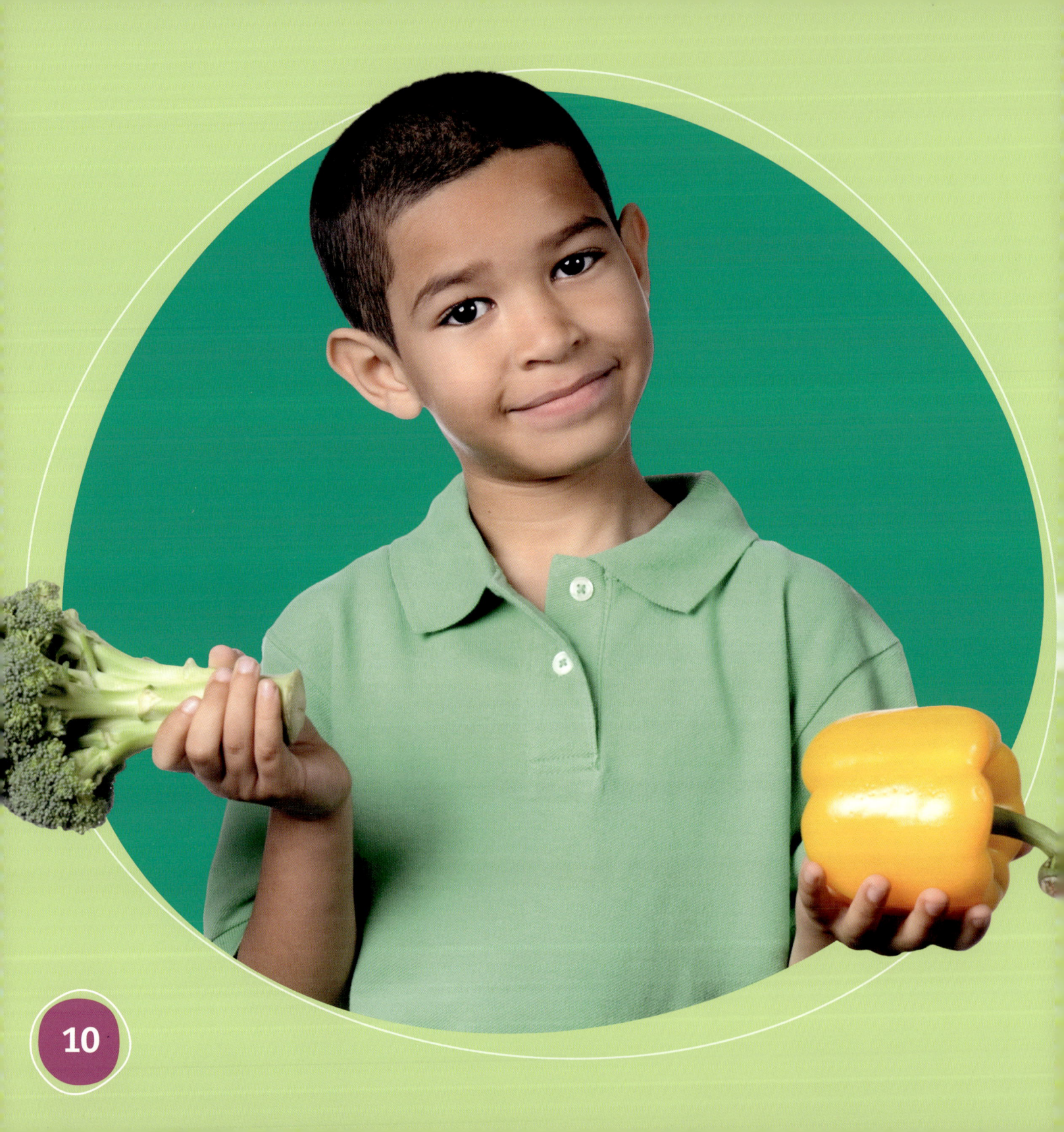

Get vitamin C from broccoli and bell peppers.

Vitamin C helps cuts heal.

Some vegetables are starchy.

They give you energy.

Two of these are potatoes and corn.

What do you use energy for?

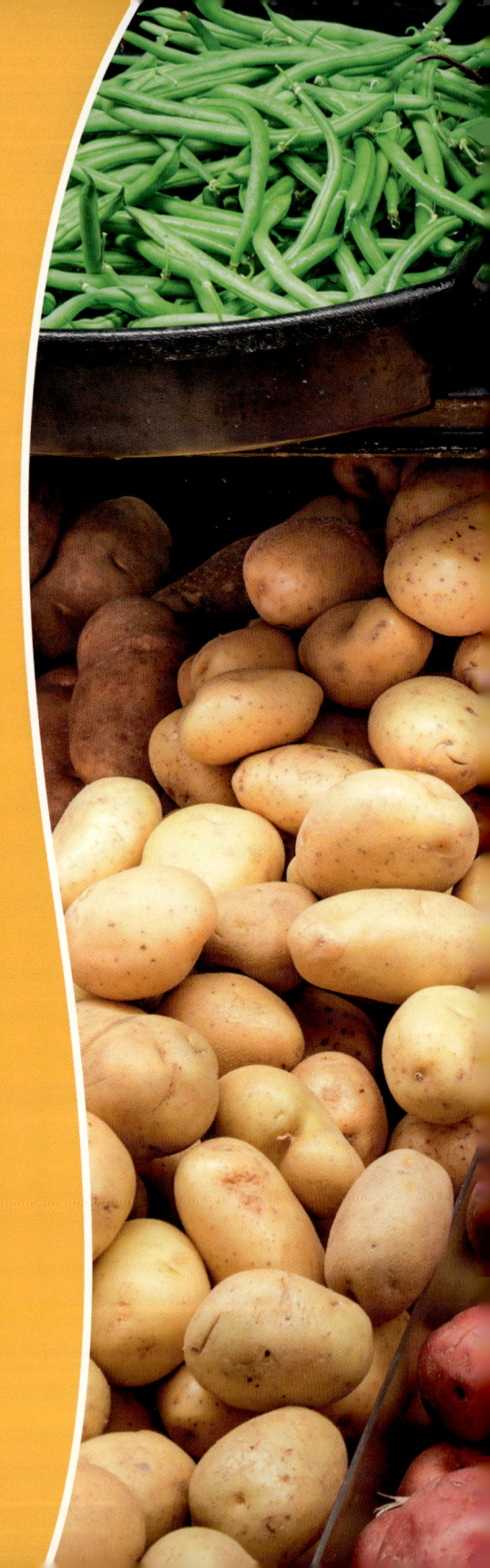

13

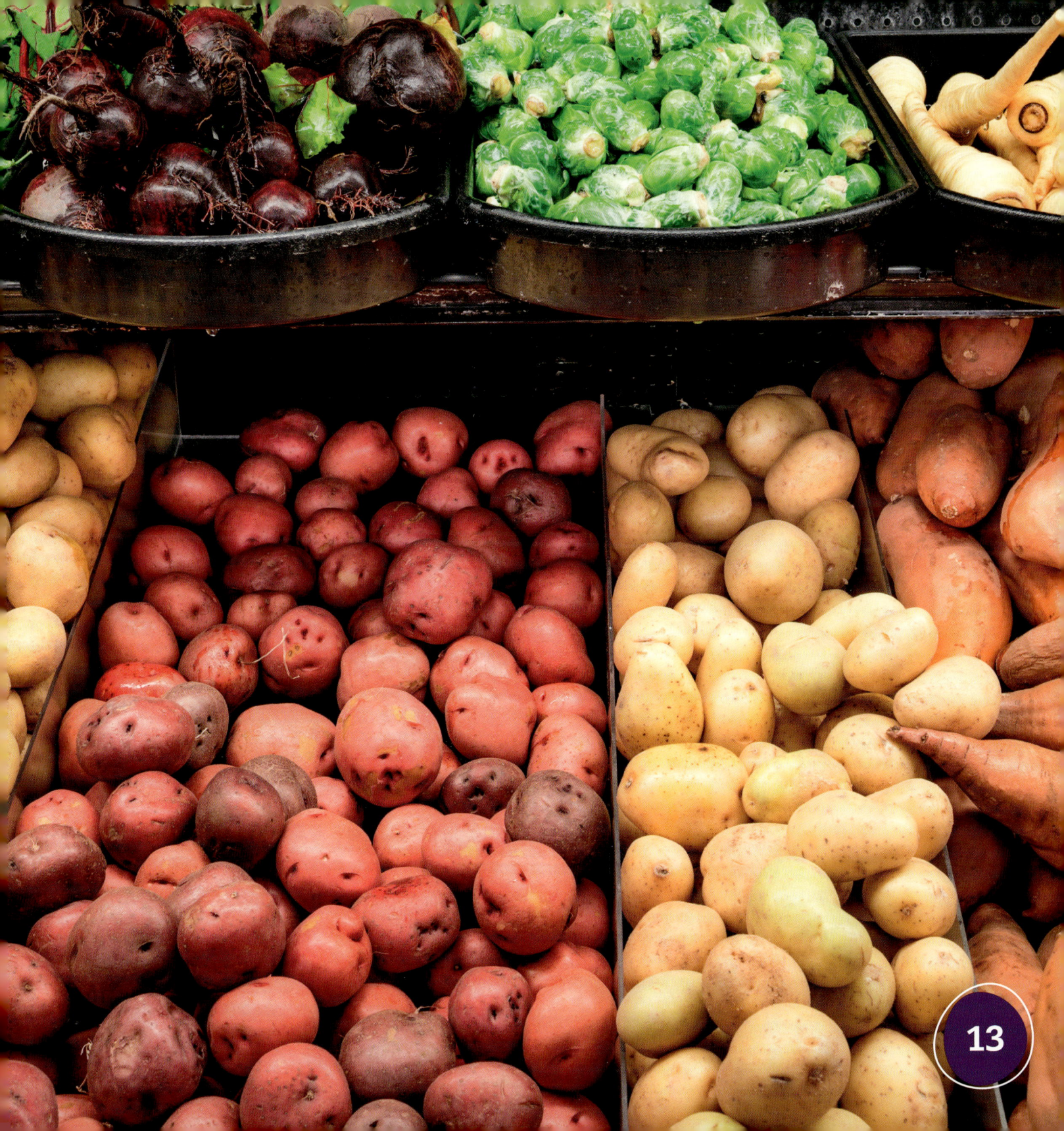

14

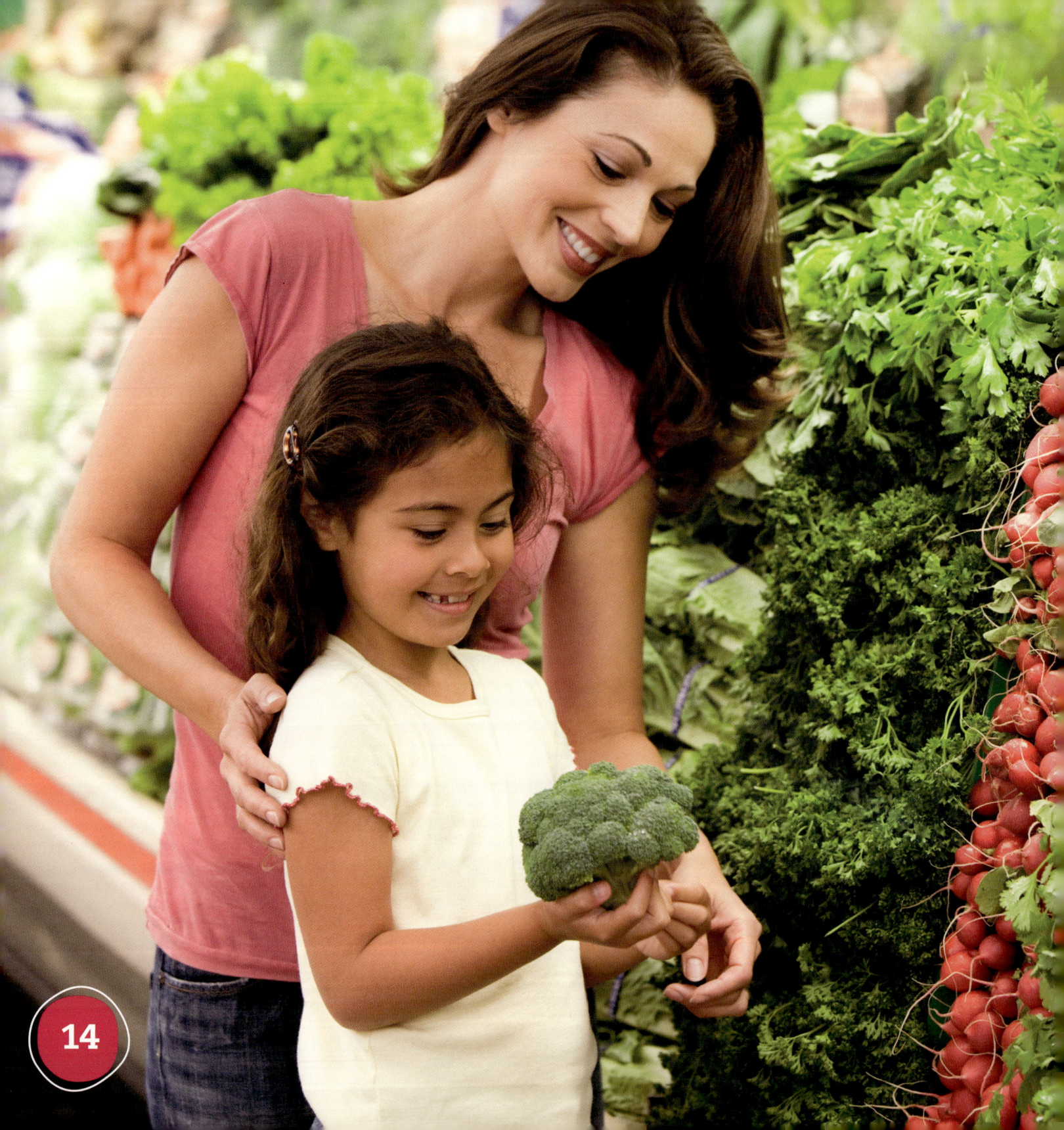

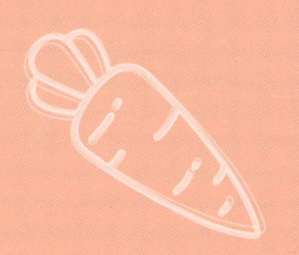

Vegetables have fiber.

Fiber helps digestion.

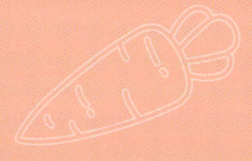

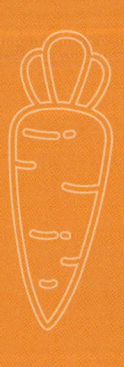

Beans have lots of fiber.

They help you feel full.

What other foods make you feel full?

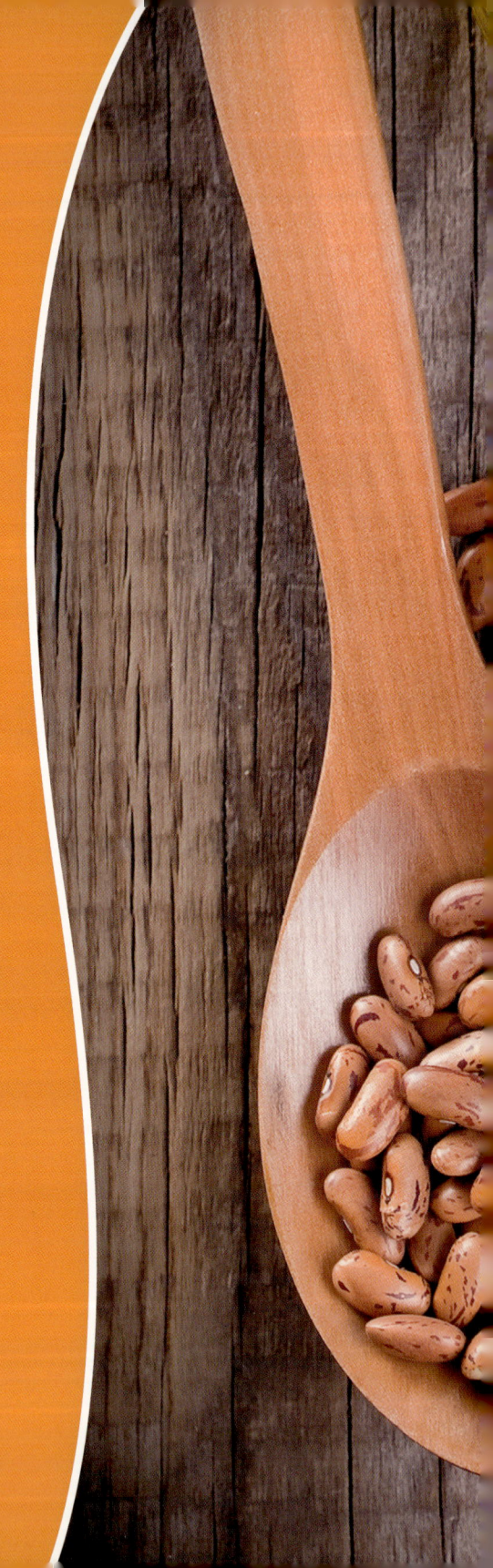

16

17

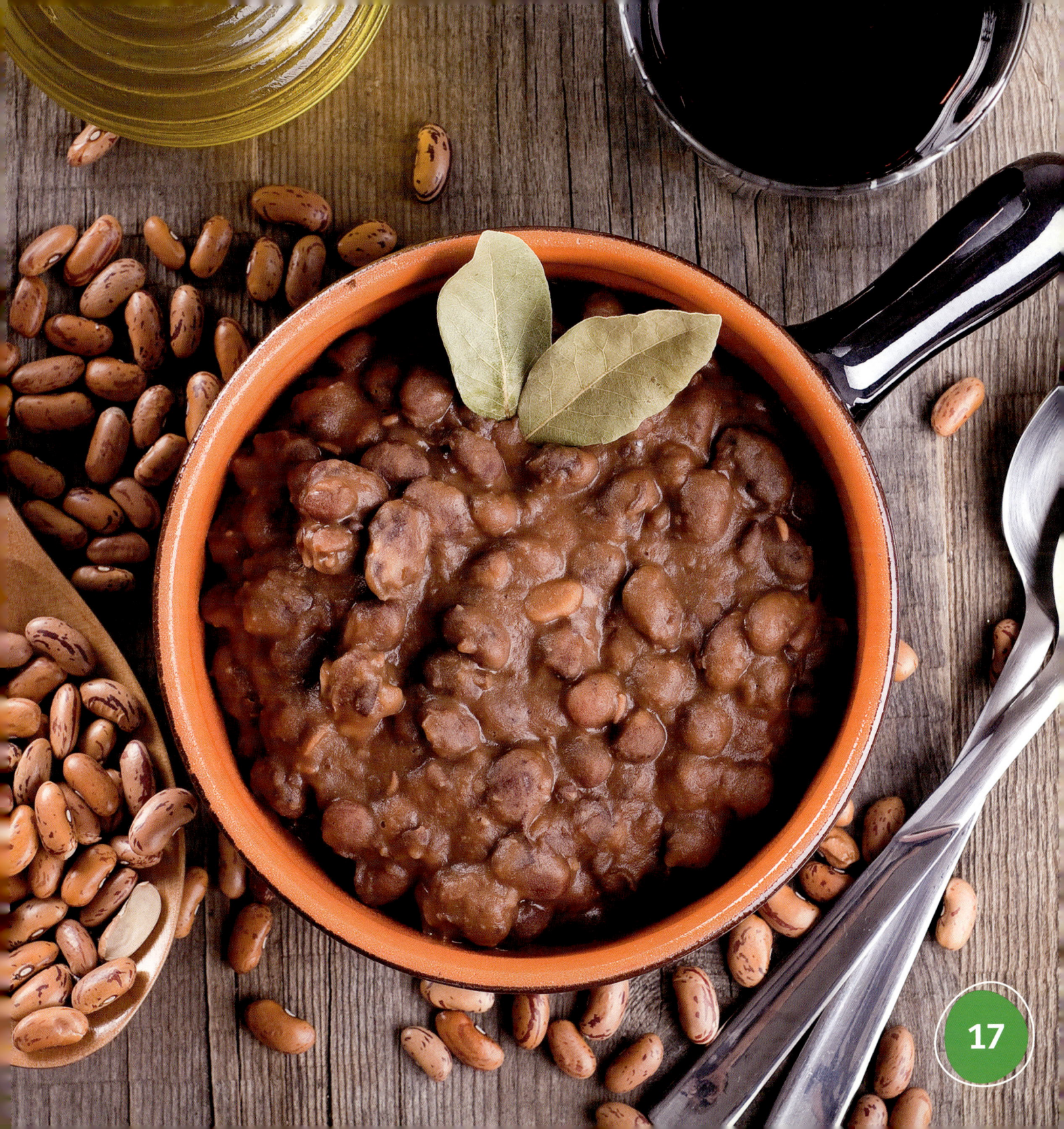

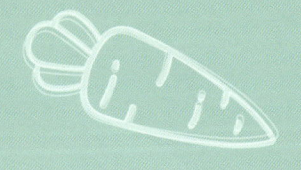

Kids need three servings of vegetables each day.

Snack on pepper slices.

Eat some carrots.

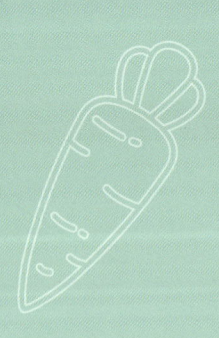

19

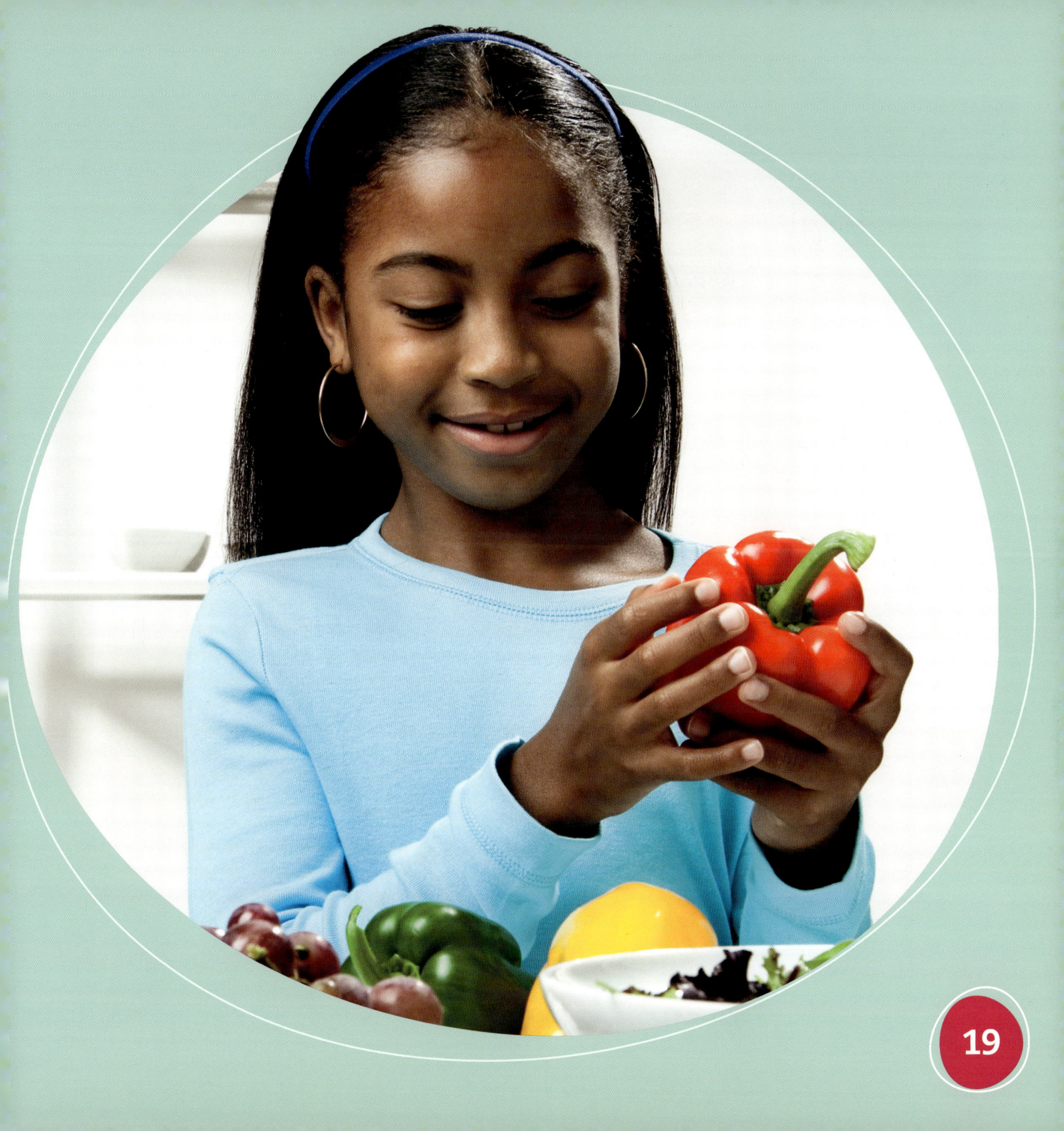

20

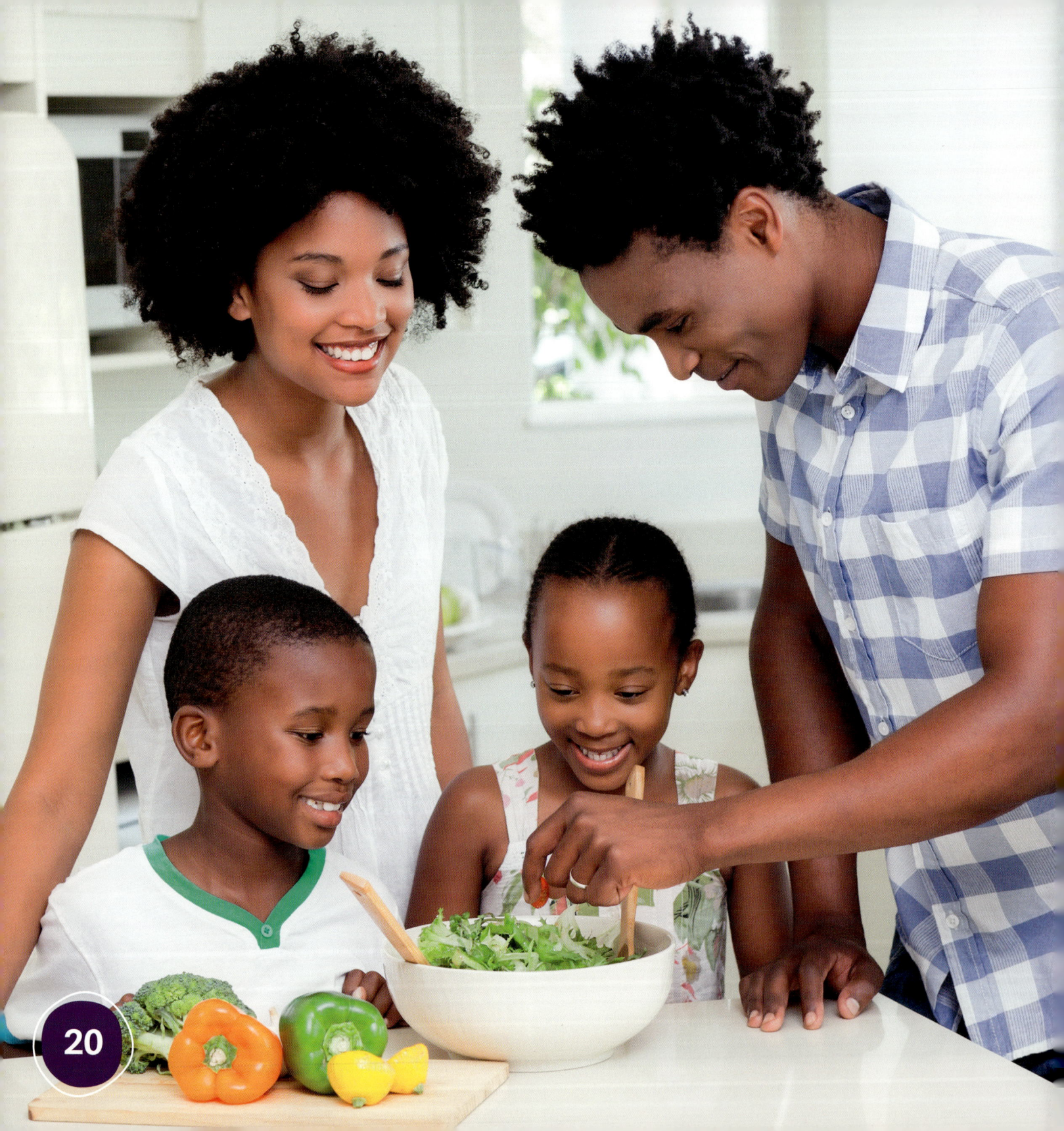

Eating vegetables helps you

stay healthy.

What are your favorite vegetables?

USDA MyPlate Diagram

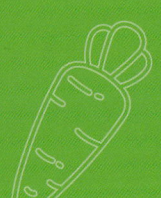

Fill this much of your plate with vegetables.

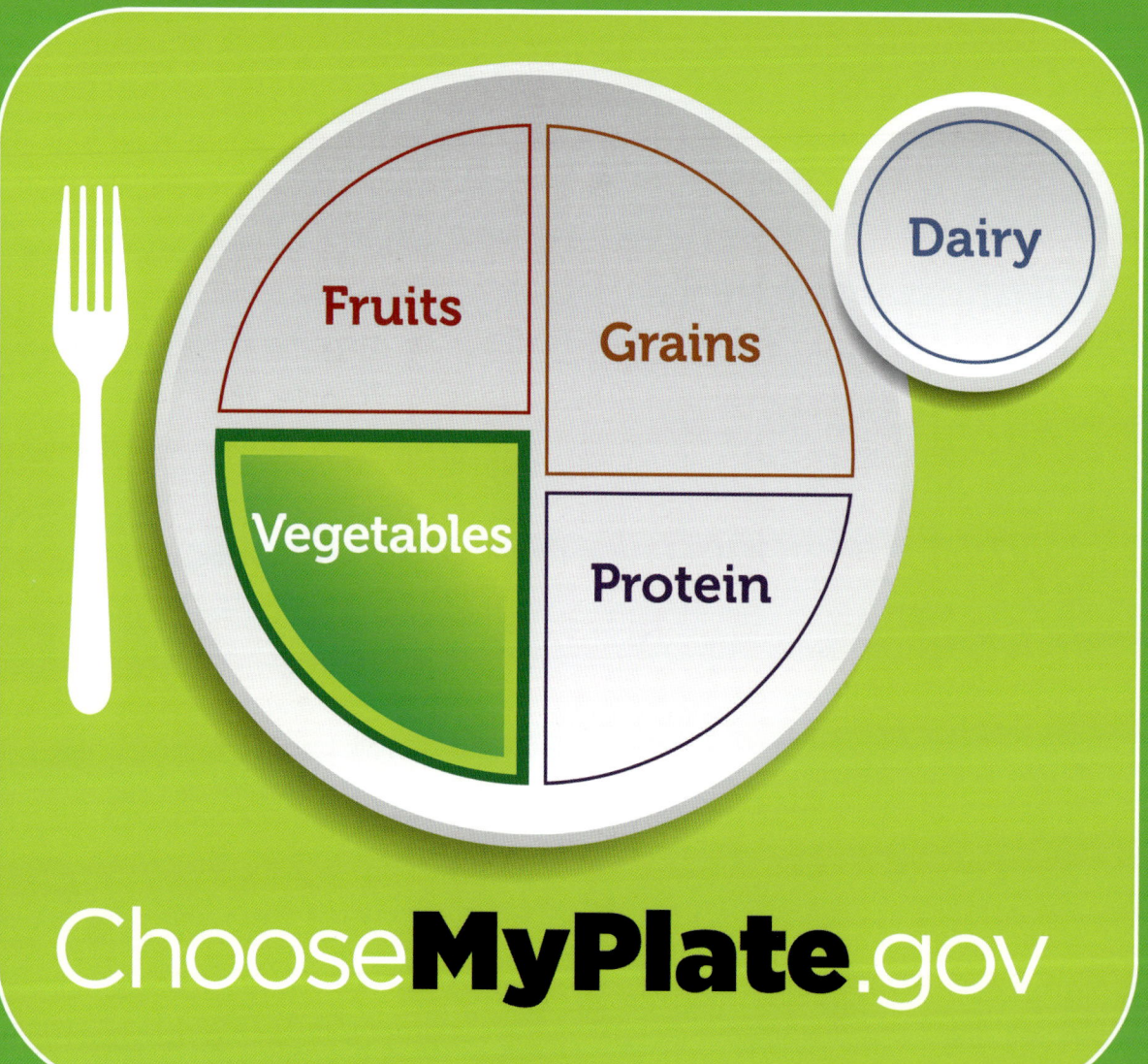

Fruits

Grains

Vegetables

Protein

Dairy

ChooseMyPlate.gov

22

Picture Glossary

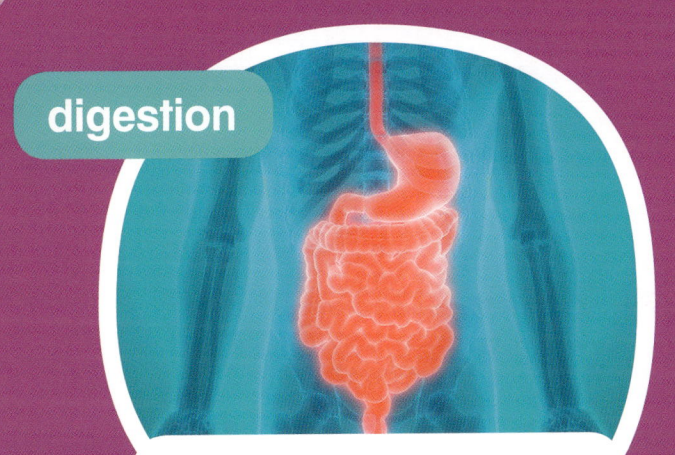

digestion
breaking down food into smaller parts the body can use

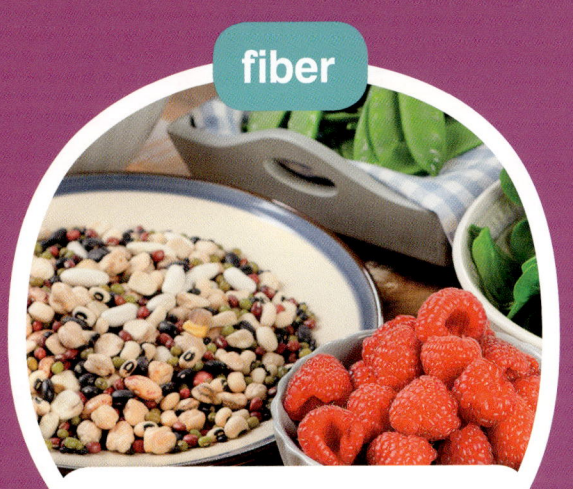

fiber
the part of plant foods that the body cannot break down

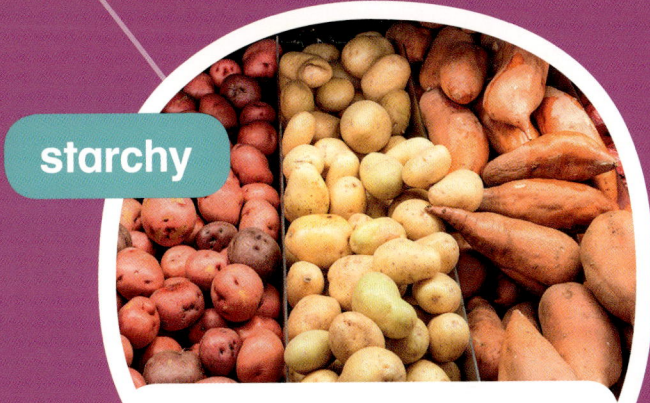

starchy
full of a substance in plants that stores energy

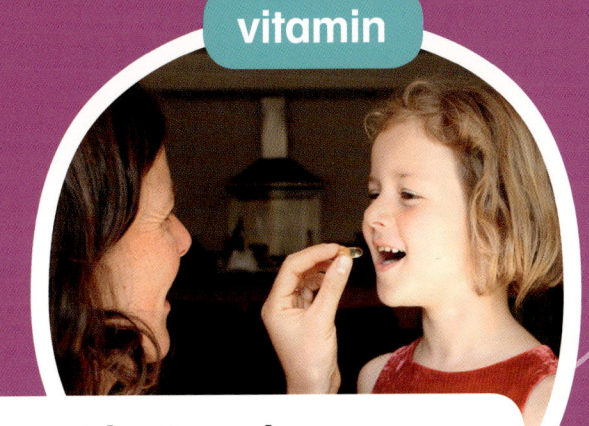

vitamin
a nutrient such as vitamin A, vitamin C, and others that your body needs for good health

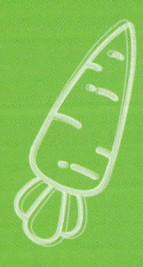

Read More

Hoffmann, Sara E. *Kinds of Vegetables*. Minneapolis: LernerClassroom, 2013.

Reinke, Beth Bence, MS, RD. *Why We Eat Fruits*. Minneapolis: Lerner Publications, 2019.

Salzmann, Mary Elizabeth. *Eat Your Vegetables! Healthy Eating Habits*. Minneapolis: Abdo, 2015.

Index

bones, 8

digestion, 15

energy, 12

fiber, 15–16

starchy, 12

vitamins, 7–8, 11

Photo Credits

The images in this book are used with the permission of: © unguryanu/Shutterstock.com, p. 5; © Monkey Business Images/Shutterstock.com, p. 6; © Svetl/iStock.com, pp. 8–9; © nicolesy/iStock.com, p. 10; © Trong Nguyen/Shutterstock.com, pp. 12–13, 23 (bottom left); © Monkey Business Images/Shutterstock.com, p. 14; © milla1974/Shutterstock.com, pp. 16–17; © Thomas_EyeDesign/iStock.com, p. 19; © wavebreakmedia/Shutterstock.com, p. 20; © US Department of Agriculture, p. 22; © Magic mine/Shutterstock.com, p. 23 (top left); © bitt24/Shutterstock.com, p. 23 (top right); © stevenrwilson/iStock.com, p. 23 (bottom right).

Front Cover: © Africa Studio/Shutterstock.com.

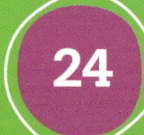